Pioneering Medicine
From Sage to Surgery

Don't Miss a Single Adventure!
Read all the books in the Fields of Silver and Gold series.

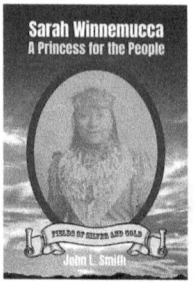

#1 Sarah Winnemucca:
A Princess for the People

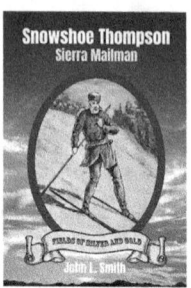

#2 Snowshoe Thompson:
Sierra Mailman

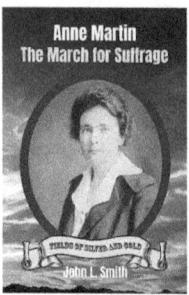

#3 Anne Martin:
The March for Suffrage

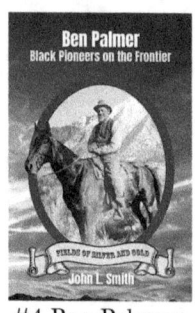

#4 Ben Palmer:
Black Pioneers on the Frontier

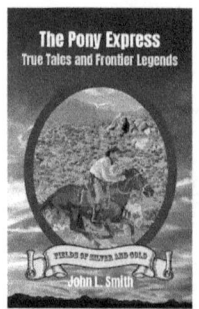

#5 The Pony Express:
True Tales and Frontier Legends

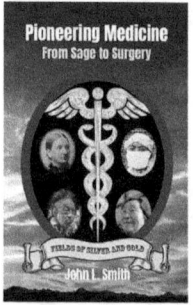

#6 Pioneering Medicine:
From Sage to Surgery

Find details at keystonecanyon.com

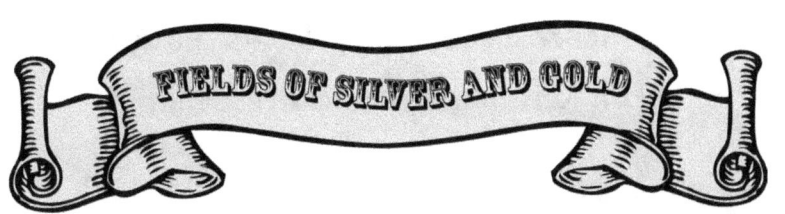

FIELDS OF SILVER AND GOLD

Pioneering Medicine
From Sage to Surgery

John L. Smith

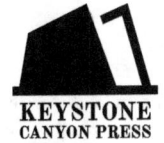

KEYSTONE CANYON PRESS

For neurosurgeon and Nevada native Dr. Kris Smith, a real lifesaver.

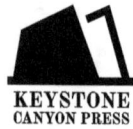

Publisher Alrica Goldstein
Copyeditor Paul Szydelko

Keystone Canyon Press
2341 Crestone Drive
Reno, NV 89523

www.keystonecanyon.com

7853886 © Igor Kolos | Dreamstime.com

Copyright © 2022 by John L. Smith

All rights reserved. No part of this book may be reproduced in any manner whatsoever without written permission except in the case of brief quotations embodied in critical articles and reviews.

Library of Congress Control Number: 2022939991

ISBN 978-1-953055-29-3
EPUB ISBN 978-1-953055-30-9

Manufactured in the United States of America

Contents

Author's Note vi
Timeline vii
1. Is There a Doctor in the Territory? 1
2. Native Healers 9
3. Chinese Medicine in the West............ 17
4. The Angels of St. Mary's: Nurses and Midwives in Early Nevada 25
5. Eliza Cook Follows Her Dream 30
6. Treating All People 38
7. Surviving the Great Influenza............ 42
8. In Pursuit of a Medical Education.......... 58
Glossary........................... 61
Key Characters...................... 62
Selected Bibliography and Further Reading... 64
Questions for Discussion 65
Index............................. 66
About the Author 69

Author's Note

Historians prefer to use primary sources (letters, diaries, speeches, and photographs) to learn about historical events. Sometimes facts aren't written down as they happen so historians use secondary sources (things written about a historical event by someone who did not witness the event). With these pieces of information, they have to be critical thinkers that put the facts that they know together to make their best guess at what really happened.

You can be a critical thinker too! Keep reading about history that makes you think and dig deeper. Find new sources and think about how that might fit in with what you already know. Understanding our history helps us understand our world.

I am grateful for all the remarkable historical research that has been invaluable to the telling of this story. In Nevada, no one has done more to archive Nevada's medical history than Dr. Anton P. Sohn. Thanks also to my friend and advocate Marydean Martin for her support. Here's to a healthier Nevada.

Timeline

1848   Gold is discovered in California near Sutter's Mill.
1849   More than 22,000 settlers pass through Carson Valley and Truckee Meadows, most on the way to California and Oregon.
1851   Dr. Charles Daggett settles in in the Carson Valley area, becomes recognized as the first practicing physician in the future state of Nevada.
1856   Mormon Station, founded in 1851, is renamed Genoa.
1850s   Midwife Nellie Nostrossa begins treating patients in Eureka.
1860   Pony Express mail service begins its brief but exciting history.
1860   Aurora is founded; the mining boomtown includes a prosperous Chinese community complete with practicing doctors.
1861–1865   Civil War is fought.
1864   On October 31, Nevada becomes the thirty-sixth state.
1870   Dr. Lemuel Lee arrives to practice medicine in Pioche, later moves to Carson City.
1876   St. Mary's Hospital opens in Reno.
1899   Midwife and nurse Mary Oxborrow practices in the community of Lund.
1899   Dr. Lee becomes first secretary of Nevada State Board of Medical Examiners.
1918   Influenza virus, also called the Spanish flu, rages throughout the United States and much of Europe.
1922   St. Mary's Hospital Training School for nurses closes.

1947 Seven intrepid Dominican Catholic Sisters of Adrian, Michigan, move to Henderson to take over the ownership, management, and care of the former Basic Magnesium Hospital, which is renamed Rose de Lima Hospital.
1969 University of Nevada School of Medicine established in Reno.
1973 Nevada Legislature passes a bill legalizing the ancient Chinese medical practice of acupuncture, making the state the first in the nation to do so.
2014 The UNLV School of Medicine is established with Dr. Barbara Atkinson as its founding dean. It graduated its first class and was renamed the Kirk Kerkorian School of Medicine in 2021.

1
Is There a Doctor in the Territory?

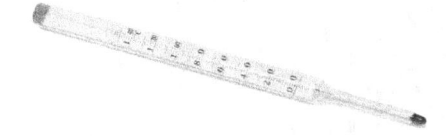

On Nevada's early frontier, few men rivaled Orson Hyde's influence. In 1855, he was appointed judge and leader of the Utah Territory, out of which Nevada would one day be carved. He was also a high official of the Church of Jesus Christ of Latter-day Saints, which had sent some of its members from Salt Lake City to settle in the Carson Valley in the early 1850s at a time when it was a part of the Utah Territory. They arrived in part to raise cattle and grow produce to sell to the growing numbers of emigrants who traveled through the valley throughout the year on their way to the gold fields of California and the Sierra Nevada range.

It was there in the mountains that Hyde found himself caught in a December snowstorm. The deadly Donner Party tragedy a decade earlier was still fresh in many minds, and miners and immigrants commonly froze to death trying to cross the unforgiving Sierra Nevada in winter.

Pressing on through the icy conditions, Hyde later recalled going without sleep for four nights and running out of food. Hyde found himself suffering from frostbitten legs and needing immediate medical

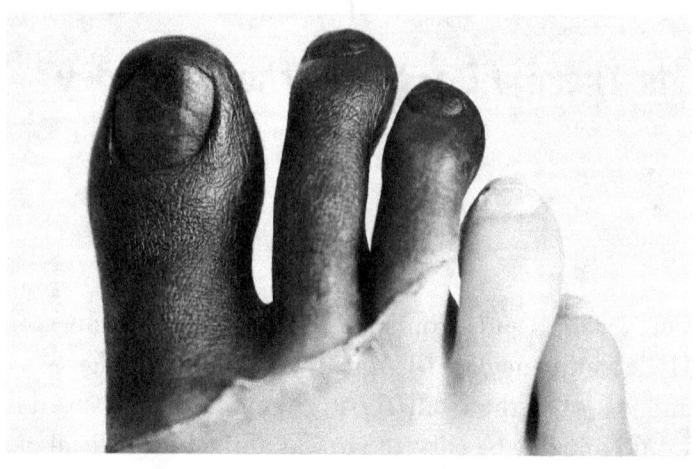

This final stage of frostbite is when the bones and tendons freeze and is irreversible. In the early stages, the skin turns white and needs treatment.

assistance. The super-cold temperature had frozen the skin of his lower legs and feet and slowed his circulation. Without emergency help, he was destined to lose his feet and perhaps even his life.

Fortunately for Hyde, he managed to make his way to the door of Dr. Charles Daggett, frontier Nevada's first practicing physician. The judge was in dire shape. There was no time to waste.

Daggett's experience had taught him that quickly warming up Hyde's feet would do more harm than good. Daggett needed to increase Hyde's blood circulation slowly, and so he took the judge to an iced-over creek near Daggett's cabin.

As reported by the judge and in future accounts by historians and journalists, Daggett first chopped an opening through the ice. He then placed Hyde's lower legs into the creek's near-freezing water. Ever so slowly, the judge's frost-darkened feet and lower legs began to thaw out.

Once the circulation returned color to his patient's extremities, Daggett was able to bring Hyde into the cabin, where he rubbed on his feet and legs a trusted mixture that included turpentine. (Turpentine is an oil extracted from pine and other trees.) After doing so, he loosely packed the judge's legs and feet in cotton.

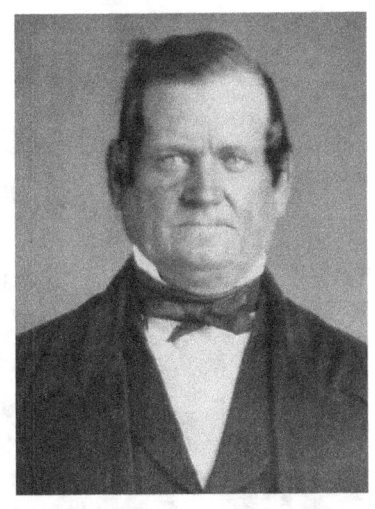

Orson Hyde was a leader in the early Latter Day Saint Church.

Hyde's legs and feet were saved without the benefit of the kind of advanced medical treatment that we take for granted today. In Daggett's time, even the best-trained medical doctors relied on treatments that mixed herbs, oils, and even animal parts to make what were little more than home remedies. Western medicine in the 1850s still had much to learn.

To a grateful Judge Hyde, however, Daggett was a medical marvel. The judge was back on his feet the next day and returned home by horse-drawn buggy. Gradually, his feet healed sufficiently to allow him to

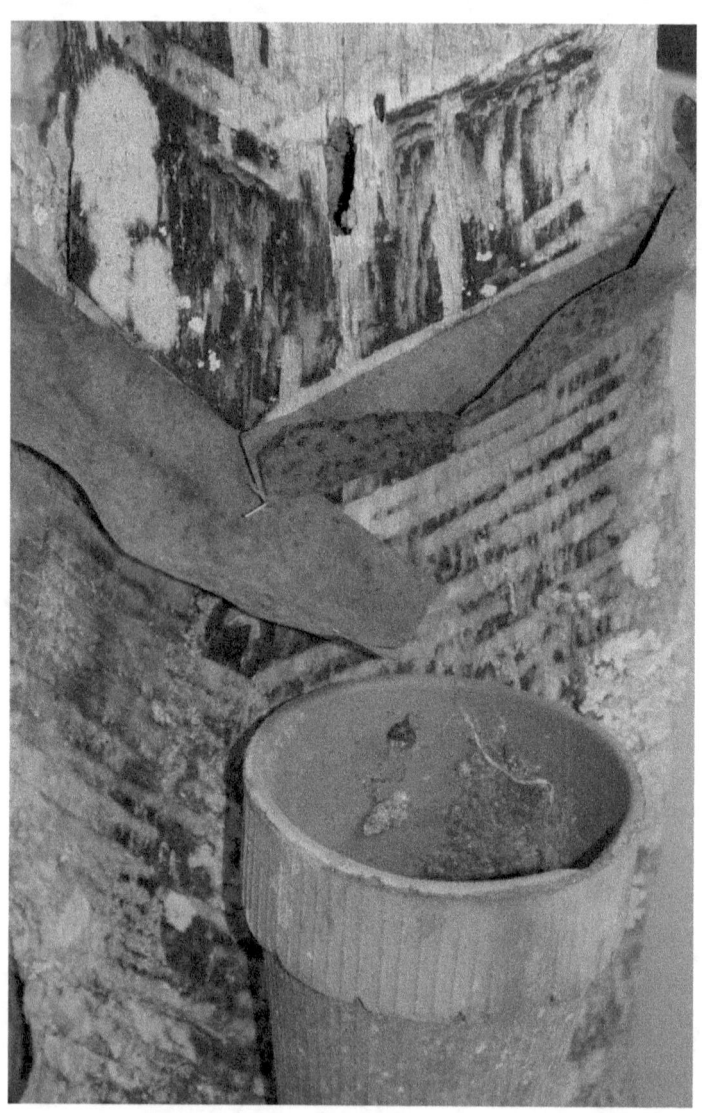

Turpentine is produced by cutting v-shaped stripes into pine trees and collecting sap that gets boiled down and used as a solvent. It was also used to kill lice, clean wounds, and relieve pain.

regain most of their use. He later wrote to the LDS Church's leader Brigham Young that "one foot now well, the other doing well, but looks like anything other than a foot."

The story of Dr. Daggett saving Judge Hyde's frozen feet is considered one of the first documented cases of medical treatment in frontier Nevada. It wouldn't be the last time Daggett's medical training came in handy. The fact that he had an actual medical education at all set him apart from many of the men and women who would call themselves doctors in Nevada's earliest days.

Daggett was born in 1806 in Vermont and educated at Berkshire Medical College in Pittsfield, Massachusetts. As with other groundbreaking acts associated with Daggett, his familiarity with the law led to him becoming Nevada's first resident attorney. He served as the county prosecutor of persons accused of committing crimes and acted as the county tax collector. He also played an integral role in the creation of Nevada's statehood in 1864.

Daggett was the first of many physicians who came to the Nevada frontier to practice medicine, but his presence was not without controversy. It has also been reported that he arrived in Carson Valley in possession of two African American slaves, who later won their freedom.

An astute businessman, Daggett looked at the Georgetown Trail that linked to a pass that led over

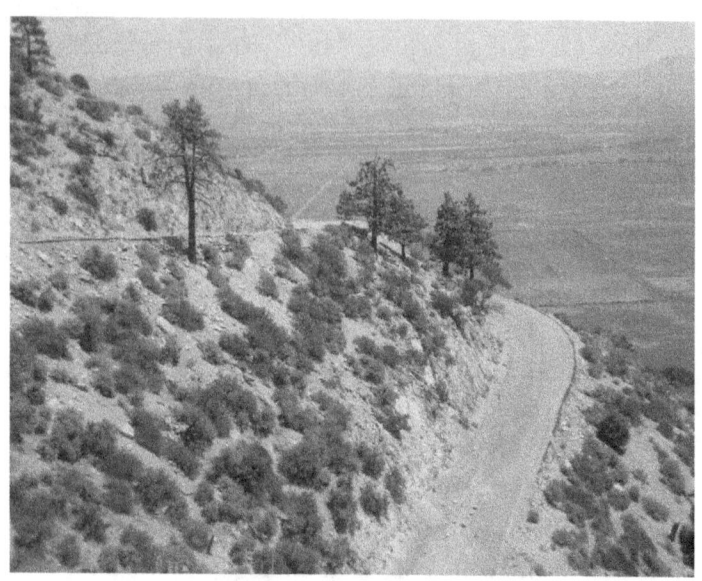

Dr. Charles Daggett purchased land at the base of the Sierra Nevada and made efforts to improve the Kingsbury Grade over the pass so that wagons could manage it as well as mules and foot travelers.

to Lake Tahoe and saw an opportunity. He purchased the land at the base of the road. It later came in handy when David Kingsbury and John McDonald obtained the rights to build a toll road up and over the steep mountain. It was christened the Kingsbury Grade, and Daggett Pass was named for the doctor, who also put his name on a nearby creek.

But to better appreciate Daggett as a doctor, it is helpful to remember that much of what we now take for granted in medicine—even simple treatments such as aspirin for a headache, or an elastic bandage for a wrist sprain—had not yet been developed or were

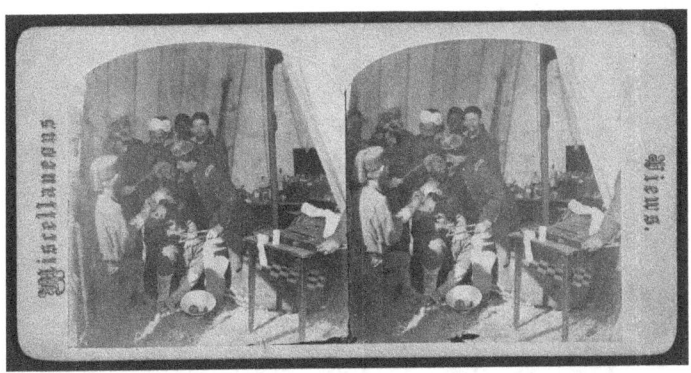

Stereoscopic photos were first exhibited in 1851. The photographer takes two copies of the same view set about 2.5 inches apart. By taking the images at slightly different angles, the viewer gets a 3D sense of the scene, like this one of a Civil War amputation.

not in wide use. (Aspirin was first developed in 1897, the elastic bandage in 1914.) That was especially true on the frontier of the West, where even crude general stores were few and far between.

It is important to understand that Americans, as a whole, live much longer today than they did back in 1850. The average life expectancy in frontier Nevada was about thirty-nine years. Thanks in great part to advancements in medicine, physician training, science, healthcare, and nutrition, today Americans live an average of seventy-eight years.

Life was difficult. Death during childbirth was common. Diseases such as influenza, scarlet fever, typhoid fever, tuberculosis, and even the measles were highly contagious and considered deadly. Little was understood about germs and viruses. In a time before

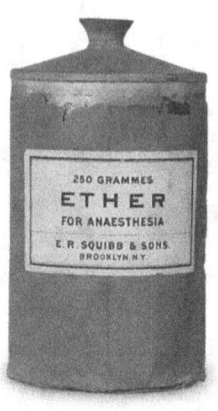

Ether was developed as an early anaesthetic in 1842 and continued to be regularly used until the 1960s.

the development of vaccines and other medicines that today we take for granted, even the common cold took many lives.

Before the creation of educational standards and medical certification, doctors arrived in Nevada with widely varied skills. Some were just barbers who, in addition to cutting hair, also offered "medical" opinions about everything from broken bones to sudden fevers. Some sold *patent medicine* that was often little more than alcohol and included traces of the powerful natural painkiller opium. And after the American Civil War (1861–1865), a new generation of physicians and nurses who arrived in the West were accustomed to seeing and attempting to treat the horrifying damage inflicted during battle.

Although historians generally agree that Daggett was the first medically educated doctor to treat patients in the place that would one day be called the state of Nevada, he was far from the only healer in the land.

2

Native Healers

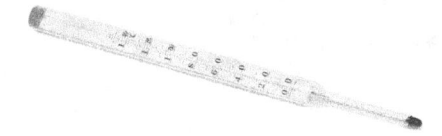

While Charles Daggett is credited as Nevada's first physician, that just depends on your definition of "doctor." By the time Daggett arrived in the Carson Valley, Native American healers had been roaming the Sierra Nevada and Great Basin for hundreds of years treating the physical, mental, and spiritual ailments of the Paiute, Shoshone, Washoe, and other indigenous tribes.

Unlike many conventional physicians, the Native American healers combined vast knowledge of the medicinal properties of plants and minerals with rituals and ceremonies passed down through generations. Plants, roots, and herbs were used to treat illness, and spiritual health played an important role in the process.

Individual tribes often had their own distinct healing practices and rituals. Many tribes based their philosophy of the treatment of illness on the *medicine wheel* or *medicine hoop* that symbolized the connection of the people physically and spiritually to the earth. Four cardinal directions—north, south, east, and west—were represented on the wheel along with the sky above,

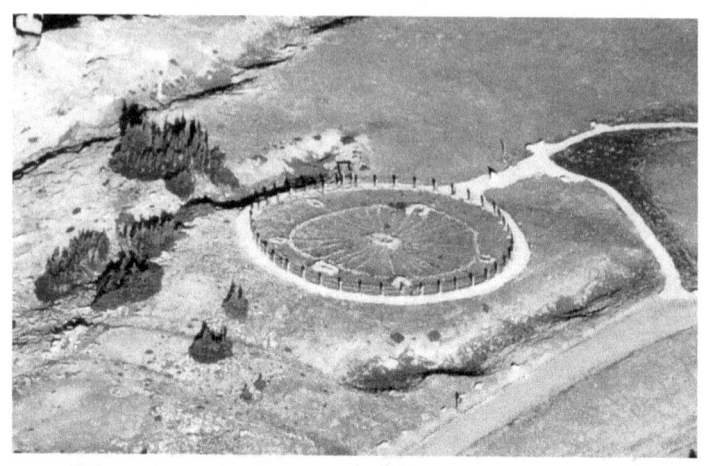

The medicine wheel in Bighorn National Park, Wyoming is both a place of sacred ceremony and scientific inquiry. It is eighty feet in diameter.

the earth below, and the spirit of the living tree in the center. In addition to their physical uses, plants and animals had spiritual meanings for tribes as well.

In their way, tribal remedies were sometimes like those used by early settlers. In the time before modern medicine, herbs and leaves were sometimes boiled and made into medicinal teas. Wounds were sometimes treated with a poultice, moist plant material or even flour that was then wrapped in cloth.

Native healers also made use of the available natural waters to treat illness. The medicinal properties of the mineralized water of hot springs that bubbled up from underground was an effective treatment for the pain of sore muscles and aching bones. Think of it as a frontier hot tub!

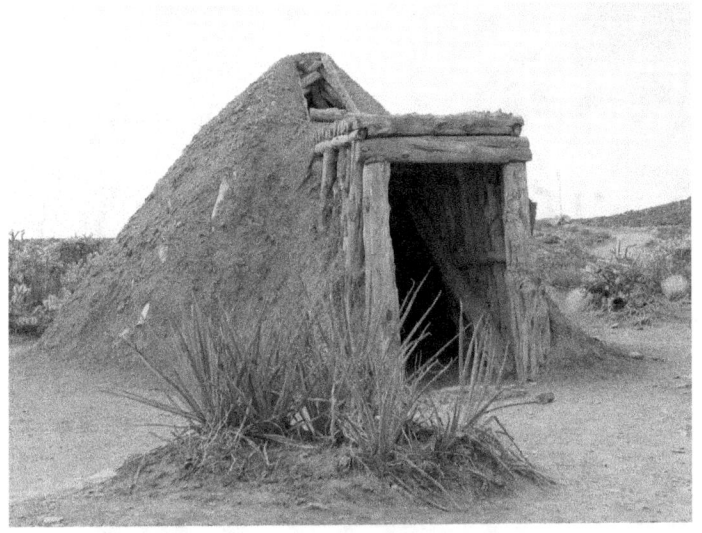

Sweat lodges like this one were used as a way to purify the mind and body to cure illness.

The ill were sometimes sent to a sweat lodge to break a fever or remove impurities through perspiration. The lodge was often a humble tent structure heated by hot stones that raised the air temperature high enough to enable those inside to break a sweat. Long before saunas became popular, there was the sweat lodge.

Native treatments sometimes included the use of crystals, healing stones, "medicine bags" carried to heal and ward off sickness, prayers, chants, dances, and meditative walks.

A healer called a shaman was considered a doctor and spiritual leader in many tribes. He held a position of importance, but with that trust came great responsibility.

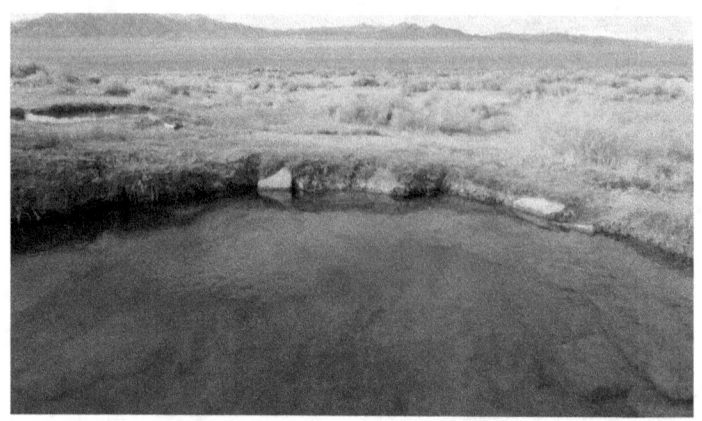

Hot springs like this one at Ruby Valley Refuge bubble up throughout Nevada and can be enjoyed by people even today.

The history of some tribes includes instances in which a shaman who failed to heal a patient, or refused someone treatment, was put to death.

For a moment, imagine taking a walk with a native healer on the frontier. The vast desert stretches for miles around before it reaches the distant mountains dotted with pine and juniper trees. Across the valley, steam rises from a natural hot spring.

In the low desert, the humble greasewood bush, also called a creosote bush, has tiny leaves that feel oily to the touch—a sign that it is a plant growing in an area that receives scant rainfall. No matter. Native healers and frontier settlers have long used its leaves in a medicinal tea.

On this walk, you pass a mesquite tree. Its wood is hard, and it provides little shade, but the native healer knows its bark can be used to treat stomach ailments

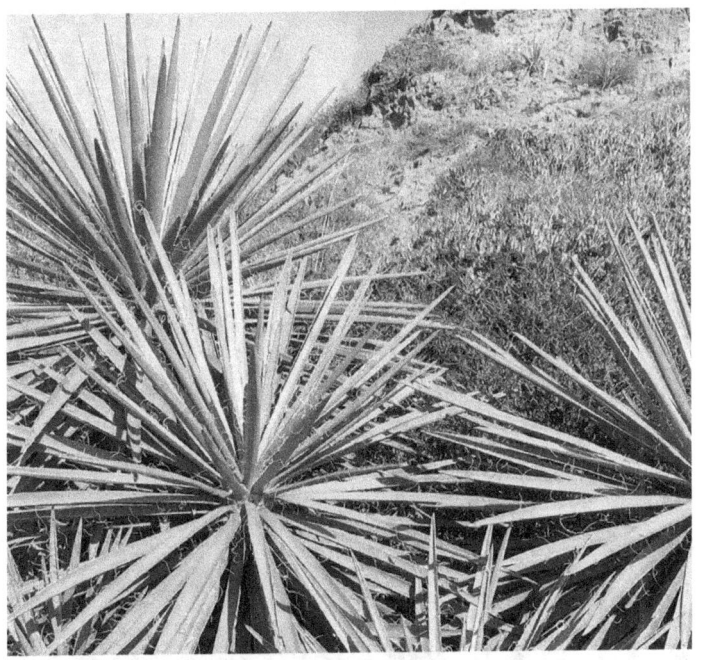

Yucca, which is easy to grow in full sun, can be used to boost the immune system and treat headaches and arthritis.

and indigestion. When processed by experienced hands, its sap can help cleanse wounds, treat sore throats, and care for many other ailments.

Over there, a yucca plant has taken hold in the desert soil. It looks spiny and unappealing, but the root can be made into soap and has other useful purposes.

Along the wash, where water flows during rainstorms and after the spring snowmelt, the willow's bright green leaves are visible. Those leaves can be made into a poultice to treat skin infection. Some people use

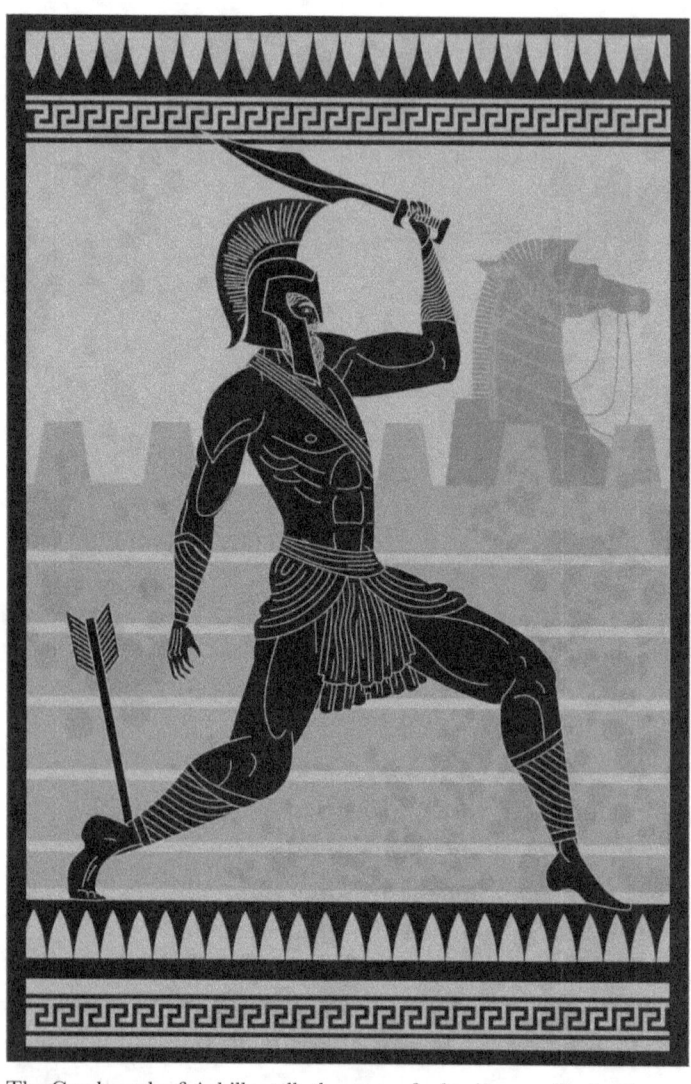

The Greek myth of Achilles tells the story of a boy's mom dipping the boy into the rivery Styx to make him invincible. She held him by his heel which became the one place he was vulnerable (Achilles' heel).

willow leaves in the right mixture as a pain reliever.

As you walk on through the desert toward the foothills, you pass a prickly pear cactus. Its spines are needle-sharp, but inside it possesses medicinal properties that trained healers have long used to treat burns and wounds. Its remarkable healing power continues to be discovered even in modern times.

And everywhere around is sage, which smells so fragrant after a rain. Some tribal healers will burn it to cleanse the body of negative spiritual energy. Others will use parts of it to treat cuts and even colds and flu.

Walk even more and you reach the marshland near the shores of Washoe Lake and Pyramid Lake. There the tall grasses and cattails have many uses from clothing to baskets, and even food. In trained hands, they are also used to treat burns, bee stings, and wounds. They have cleansing properties that aid in wound care, and their tender parts produce a sap-like substance that can help numb a toothache.

At last, you reach the foothills, where the terrain steepens, the plant life is greener, the weather cooler, and the sound of a trickling creek is heard. The wild mint and rose by the creek are used in tea to treat colds and indigestion, among other things.

At higher altitude, the trained healer uses the flowering yarrow to stop bleeding in a treatment that crosses cultures and continents. It has been written that the great Achilles of Greek mythology used yarrow on his battle wounds. Other cultures around the world

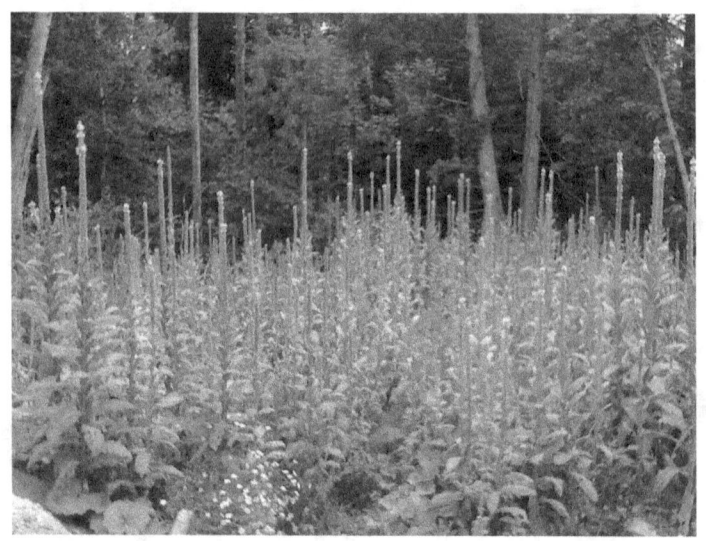

Mullein will grow in almost any open space including abandoned lots.

have used it similarly. Yarrow is also boiled into tea to reduce inflammation and inprove digestion.

The list goes on and on. Plants and herbs of all kinds have been used for centuries for medicinal purposes by those who understand their healing powers.

For one last example, let's use the mullein plant, which is sometimes called the "velvet plant" because of its fuzzy, green surface and "elephant's ear" because of its shape. It has been used for centuries for any number of ailments but is prized as a treatment for blisters and infection because of its softness.

On ranches throughout Nevada and much of the West, mullein had gained yet another nickname: "Cowboy Bandages."

3

Chinese Medicine in the West

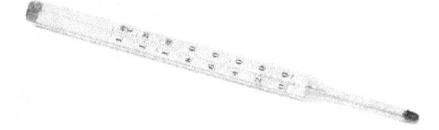

The native people weren't the only ones to use plants and herbs for healing. The search for gold and silver in Nevada and California generated an unprecedented migration to the West. Most of the fortune seekers, about 80 percent, traveled across country from the East in wagon trains, on horseback, and even on foot. Some arrived by ship all the way from China, more than 6,500 miles, ending their journey in bustling San Francisco.

Before 1848, only about fifty Chinese people lived in America, then a nation of about twenty-three million. That all began to change at the end of the decade, and by 1853 about 24,000 Chinese had made the long trip to the continent. Traditional Chinese Medicine relied on herbal treatments and practices that were sometimes thousands of years old.

Most of the first arrivals were men who, having heard of the riches to be made in America, traveled to work in the fields of silver and gold. The Chinese brought a strong work ethic and their own customs, cultural traditions, language—and medical practices, some far older than those that existed on the frontier.

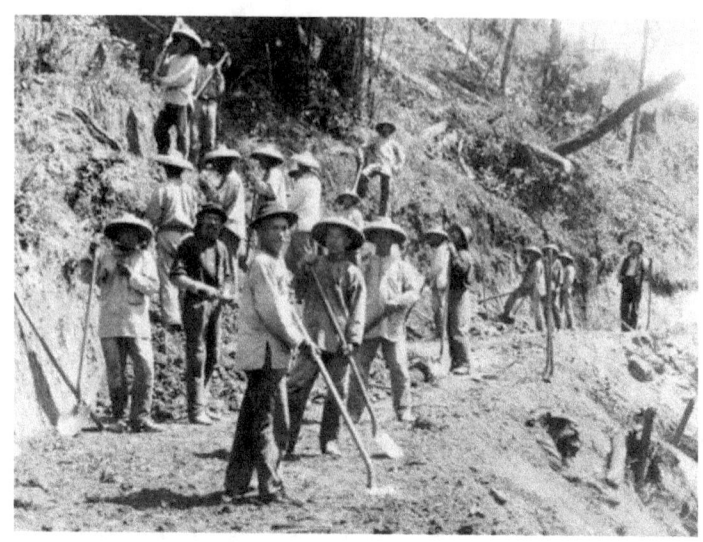

Between 1863 and 1869, roughly fifteen thousand Chinese worked on the transcontinental railroad living in tents while white workers lived in train cars. They were paid less than whites and required to work the most dangerous jobs but their tradition of boiling water for hot tea kept them from getting sick from water-born illnesses.

From the start Chinese immigrants faced racial discrimination and segregation from white society. They were deprived of civil rights, could not vote, could not testify in court, and could not become citizens.

Although their numbers weren't large outside of San Francisco, their presence in California resulted in the 1852 passage of a monthly tax on all foreign miners. The tax generated millions of dollars for California but did not protect the Chinese from racially motivated violence.

Still, they endured and managed to prosper as America moved West. After the passage of the Pacific

Railway Acts of 1862 and 1864, large railroad projects began that used thousands of Chinese laborers who were willing to work longer hours for lower wages. Even the harshest conditions in America offered a better life than most experienced in China.

Before Nevada's statehood, its Chinese population was quite small. Just twenty-three were counted in the 1860 census. As the need for mining and railroad labor grew over the next two decades, the state's Chinese population rose to 5,416 (8.7 percent of a total of 62,266).

Although relatively little was written in the newspapers about Chinese physicians in early Nevada, as early as 1870 many of them registered as doctors in the state and located their practices in Virginia City, Carson City, Reno, and Eureka. Occasionally doctors with exotic-sounding names such as Ack Sue Tong, Che Chung Hing, Hy Yick Chu, and Wong Quong were highlighted in the newspapers.

While railroads needed building and mines were prospering, the Chinese found lots of work, much of it dangerous. More than one hundred Chinese laborers were killed in a single avalanche in the Sierra Nevada during the construction of the Central Pacific Railroad. From 1863 to 1869, almost fifteen thousand Chinese workers assembled to help construct the transcontinental railroad.

Although they were often segregated from white residents, some Chinese made homes in the mining towns that sprung up throughout Nevada's early years following the discovery of gold or silver. They opened restaurants, laundries, and even doctor's offices. One Nevada town with a prosperous Chinese population was Aurora.

Located in the west-central part of the state three miles from the Nevada-California state line, Aurora was founded in 1860. It was a wild place, and violence was common. Newspapers report Chinese lived in Aurora from its earliest days and mentioned the "Chinatown" neighborhood that included residences, laundry service, and at least one doctor.

In part because of the language barrier that existed and the coverage by newspaper reporters that reflected the common prejudices of the time, relatively little has been recorded about the day-to-day lives of Chinese immigrants. As time went on, however, the *Esmeralda Herald* and other newspapers enthusiastically reported the colorful "Chinese New Year" celebrations of their exotic neighbors.

Aurora's Chinese Gardens were also locally famous for their abundance despite rocky soil and unpredictable weather. The vegetables the gardens produced fed the entire community and beyond with radishes, onions, lettuce, cabbages, and more. The care taken by the Chinese to protect the gardens even in cold weather was noticed in the local newspapers. In time, newspapers as far away as Sacramento wrote articles about the impressive gardens of Aurora.

Although never a large percentage of the population, Chinese residents made their mark in

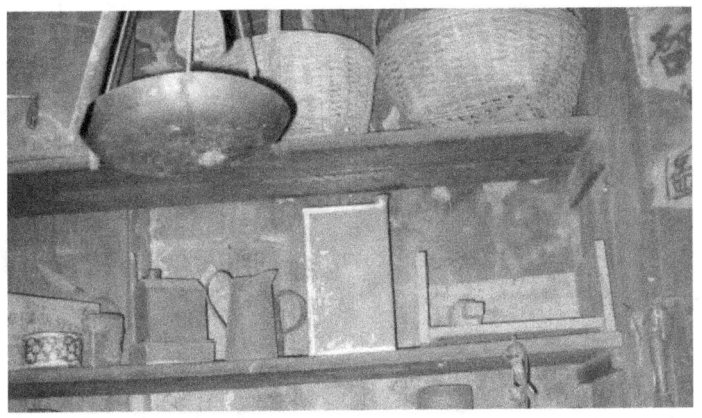

Scales, baskets for winnowing herbs, and containers were important tools for the Chinese people in the mid-1800s.

Aurora and contributed to the community despite experiencing discriminatory laws and common prejudices. As archaeologist Emily Dale observed in her study of the Chinese of Aurora that "the Chinese played an important role in Aurora's economy, both through their purchase of goods and services, and also by providing goods and services to their fellow Aurorans themselves." She concludes that "the history of the Chinese in Aurora is a complicated one."

In Aurora and elsewhere in the West, Traditional Chinese Medicine was practiced in the immigrant community. Its rich and remarkable history goes back centuries. The herbal doctors combined their knowledge of plants, minerals, and animal parts with training based on thousands of years of experimentation and observation. Compared to the

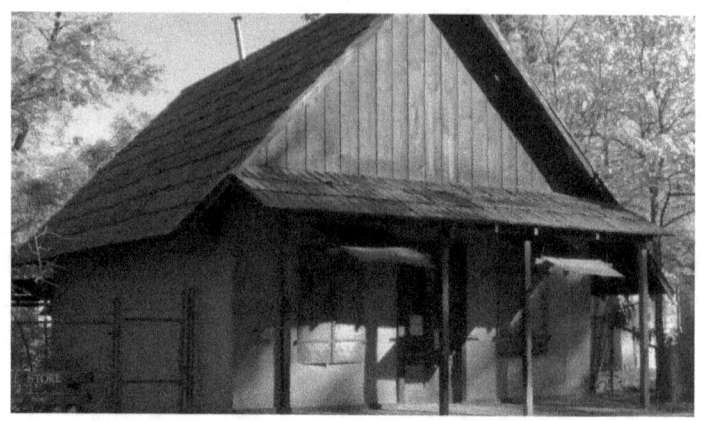

Chinese people lived and worked in the Chew Kee Store for over one hundred years tending to the needs of their community.

relatively crude medical practices of the physicians who practiced Western medicine, the Chinese doctors' treatment was very advanced. They treated not only their own people, but also white settlers as well.

Like so much of frontier Nevada, most of the buildings and streets that once housed the early Chinese community and its doctors have been lost to time. But remnants are present throughout the Sierra Nevada Gold Country, and a Chinese herbal store in Fiddletown, California, about 130 miles from Reno, is particularly well preserved. Built in 1850 of a thick clay mixture called adobe, it is named the Chew Kee Herbal Medicine Store.

Operated by Yee Fung Cheung, who was a highly respected herbal doctor, the Chew Kee Store was so successful that he opened similar stores in Virginia

City and Sacramento. Dr. Cheung gained a level of fame after he successfully treated Jane Stanford, wife of California governor Leland Stanford, for a lung ailment.

After being fully restored, the Chew Kee Store was placed on the National Register of Historic Places. Tourists and medical students today visit the store to better understand the era when Dr. Cheung operated it.

More controversially, many Chinese herbal doctors were also known to distribute the drug opium to suffering patients. Opium is highly addictive.

"On a more positive side," medical historian Dr. Anton Sohn observes, "many Chinese prescriptions and practices were just as effective, and in some cases had more efficacy than some of the nineteenth century drugs used by Americans on the western frontier. . . . It is clear that western medicine could profit from closer scrutiny of the ancient healing practices of the Chinese."

The Chinese in America struggled for many decades to achieve equality. That difficulty became even greater after the passage of the Chinese Exclusion Act of 1882, which halted immigration to the United States. Chinese immigrants were not eligible for citizenship until 1943 when the Magnuson Act repealed the Chinese Exclusion Act.

Although Nevadans historically were often slow to accept the Chinese as fellow citizens, the state is the site of a historic first in Chinese medicine. After much effort by Dr. Yee Kung Lok, Arthur Steinberg, and political lobbyist Jim Joyce, in 1973 the Nevada

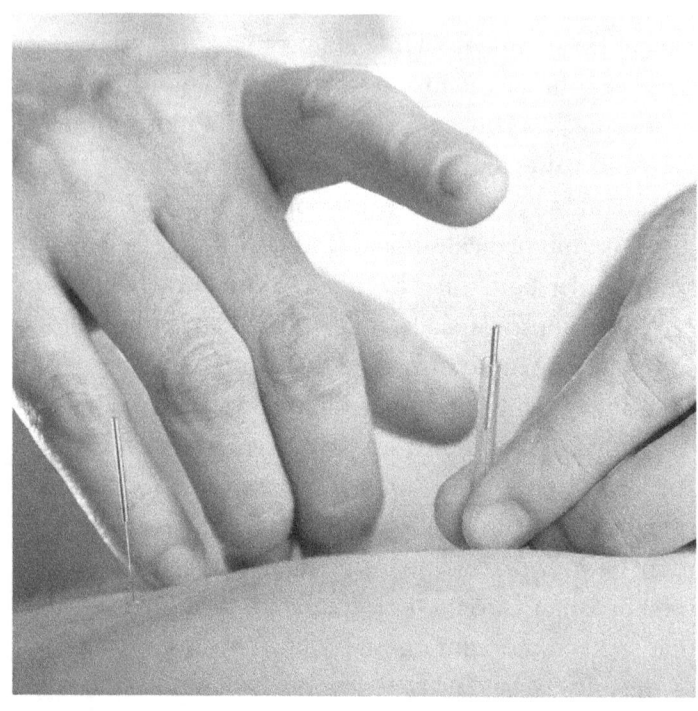

Acupuncture has been proven to manage pain and work is still being done to study what other conditions it can treat.

Legislature passed a bill making the practice of Traditional Chinese Medicine and acupuncture legal—the first US state to do so. Acupuncture is the medical procedure that uses needles to specific areas of the body to treat a wide variety of physical ailments. There are many varieties of acupuncture.

The legalization of acupuncture treatment led to the opening of medical centers as well as Wongu University of Oriental Medicine in Las Vegas.

4

The Angels of St. Mary's: Nurses and Midwives in Early Nevada

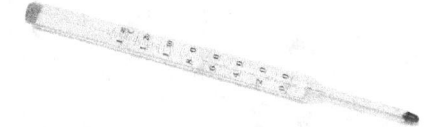

European settlers also brought their ways of treating patients and home remedies on which they relied for generations. Midwives, who are trained to assist women through pregnancy and in childbirth, and practical nurses, who are trained to care for the sick and injured and often work in hospitals, also played important roles in frontier medicine. In a time when there were few doctors, nurses and midwives with even modest medical backgrounds were highly sought after.

Early Nevada historical records indicate that during Eureka's mining boom of the late 1850s Nellie Nostrossa, a woman from Peru, received training as a midwife from two local physicians. Within a few years, other midwives and nurses received training. In 1899, Mary Oxborrow became a valuable member of the community around Lund in east-central Nevada. It is reported that she was educated as a midwife in Salt Lake City.

During the Comstock Lode mining boom of the 1860s, miners often suffered injuries, and medical care was scarce in bustling Virginia City. That began to

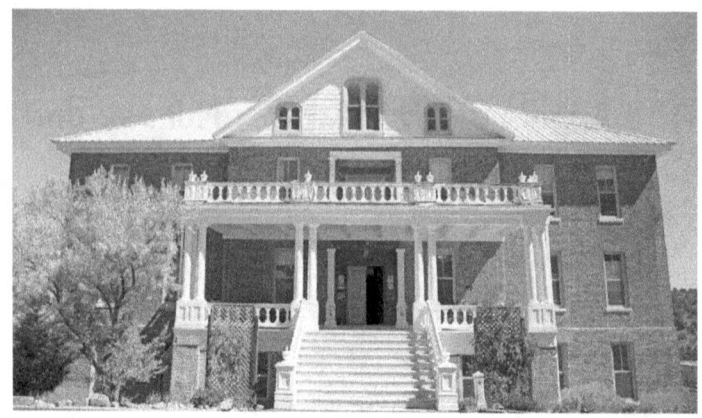

St. Mary's Hospital was built to meet the needs of the Comstock miners and served the area for decades before being converted into an art gallery.

change around the time of Nevada's 1864 statehood with the arrival of three sisters of a Catholic religious order, Mary Elizabeth, Frederica, and Xavier. They set to work to improve conditions for injured workers, families, and children in need.

On land donated by Comstock mining baron John Mackay, the Catholic sisters established St. Mary's Hospital, an impressive four-story brick building with room for up to seventy patients that opened in 1876. The hospital specialized in emergency surgery and offered the best medical care available in the state at the time.

St. Mary's Hospital of Virginia City served patients until 1940, when it closed for the next two decades. In the 1960s, a local priest and artist combined their efforts to save it from decay and demolition. It was repurposed as an arts and community center. Virginia City residents and visitors regularly gather in that historical setting to enjoy the art on display or attend a painting workshop or another of the classes offered. Those who pass through its doors invariably learn its story and its important place in Virginia City history. The sisters of St. Mary's would be proud.

By the late 1800s, nurses played an increasing role in medical care in Nevada. But without a nursing school, training them was a challenge. Attempts to train nurses in the state produced mixed results. By 1910, however, the Dominican Sisters religious order of Reno had converted a Catholic school into a hospital to accommodate the town's growing need for medical care. They also took it upon themselves to begin a school to provide nursing training in what would become a two-year program. Those who successfully completed two years were offered a third year at Sisters' Hospital, later renamed St. Mary's Hospital, as a nurse. Monthly salary: $50.

Other women received training in basic nursing by participating in the Red Cross Society of Nevada, which began with a chapter in Carson City in 1898. Groups formed throughout Northern Nevada to provide assistance to American military men serving in the Spanish-American War. They collected everything from blankets to food and clothing in a practice that would expand to include assisting families in need following natural disasters such as fires and floods.

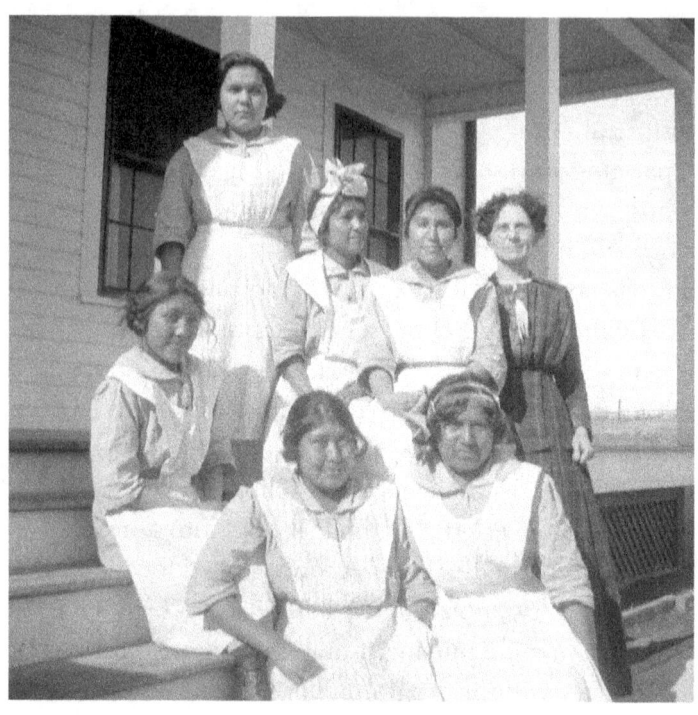

A nursing shortage in a community results in lower overall health so some communities have invested in training of their own people.

Unfortunately for Nevada, the St. Mary's Hospital Training School for Nurses closed in 1922, leaving the state without a nursing school for several decades. This created a nursing shortage that created a special hardship for rural Nevadans who lived far from the state's few large towns.

Attempts to set registration and professional standards for nurses and midwives at the Nevada Legislature began in 1915. Over the next decade, the

State Board of Nurse Examiners was established to increase the level of professionalism. A breakthrough came thanks in large part to the efforts of Assemblywoman Marguerite Gosse, who introduced the Nurse Practice Act of Nevada legislation, and Alice Craven, Mary Evans, and Emma Springmeyer as well as other members of the Nevada Nursing organization.

With each small step forward, the quality of nursing in the state improved. A more educated, professional approach was gradually replacing Nevada's wild frontier system of medical care.

Although minor training programs were created in Northern and Southern Nevada, it wasn't until 1957 that the first bachelor of science in nursing was offered at the University of Nevada, Reno. An associate degree program in nursing was developed in 1965 at the future University of Nevada, Las Vegas.

Although nursing shortages continue in modern Nevada, there is no shortage of professional training available. Nevada State College in Henderson offers a nursing program as well as UNLV and UNR. Touro University Nevada, a private institution in Henderson, offers a bachelor of science program in nursing, and the state's community colleges offer associate degree programs.

In the new century, the opportunities to pursue a career in nursing have increased along with the need for skilled professionals who choose medicine as a career path.

5

Eliza Cook Follows Her Dream

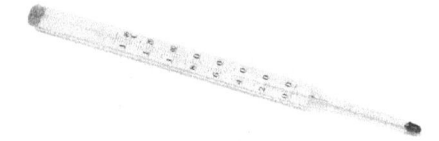

You never know where a childhood passion may take you.

Take the life story of Eliza Cook, for instance. Born in Salt Lake City in 1856, Cook developed a love of reading at an early age. She devoured story after story and reveled in the adventures she experienced as she turned the pages. Cook especially liked a tale she read about a dedicated country doctor.

After the death of her father, John, in 1870, when she was 14, Cook moved with her mother, Margaretta, and sister, Rebecca, to the Carson Valley at a time Nevada was a new state known for its boomtowns and silver and gold mines. The family settled into an area near Sheridan and Mottsville and worked to make ends meet. But the story of the helpful country physician remained with her. She dreamed that she, too, might one day become a doctor.

The very idea seemed impossible. To start, Nevada had no women physicians and few doctors at all, for that matter. It was an untamed land where even simple medical aid could be hard to find. And many of the physicians who were there lacked more than basic training. That didn't stop Cook from dreaming.

Cook put her dream into action after accepting a job in nearby Genoa at the medical office of Dr. H. W. Smith, whose wife had come down with a fever and severe abdominal pain after giving birth in the winter of 1879. Without the availability of antibiotics, which had not yet been developed, her condition was serious. She needed daily care, and Cook became her bedside companion and personal aide. In time, she made her interest in medicine known.

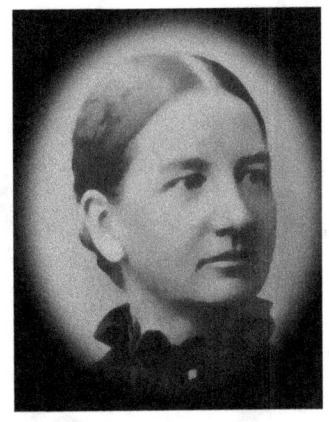

Eliza Cook, 1856-1947

As his wife recovered, Dr. Smith was so impressed by Cook's devotion that he decided to share his knowledge of medicine with her. He loaned her his medical books, gave her training, and for six months helped prepare her for the next essential step on the way to fulfilling her dream: going to medical school.

In those days, Nevada had no university medical school. The closest training was in San Francisco at Cooper Medical College, which opened in 1882 and in 1908 was renamed the Stanford University School of Medicine. With Dr. Smith's assistance, Cook enrolled and found she was one of five women in a class of sixteen students. It seemed that her dream of becoming a doctor was shared by other women.

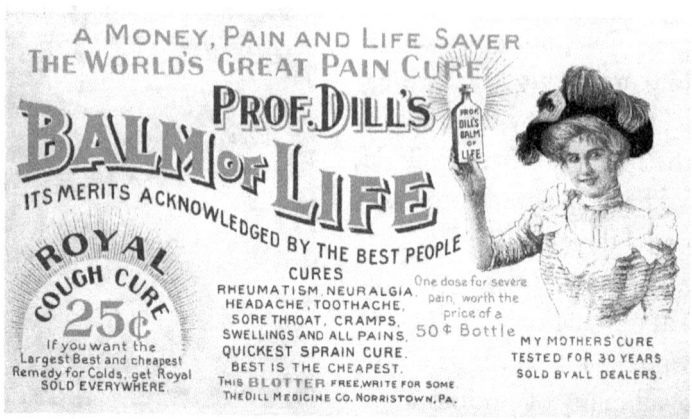

Without access to real medical care, lots of early settlers relied on cure-alls to fix whatever was ailing them. Most were primarily alcohol.

After earning her medical degree in 1884, Cook returned to Carson Valley and moved into the home owned by her sister and brother-in-law, Hugh Park. Cook managed to open a small medical practice out of the family's home, and in no time was seeing patients, most of whom were women. She traveled throughout the Carson Valley to Markleeville, California, 35 miles away.

Driving from houses and ranches in a horse-drawn buggy, for the next six years Dr. Cook practiced medicine in the region at a time of great change. She treated a wide variety of medical challenges from stitching wounds and setting broken bones to providing care for patients with potentially deadly typhoid fever. In an age before even simple aspirin was available—it was developed in 1897—ailments as common as a simple cold and flu were considered potentially fatal medical conditions.

Although Dr. Cook had come far in her medical journey, she realized there was much more to learn. In 1891, she left her practice in Nevada and enrolled at Woman's Medical College in Philadelphia, which is known as the first medical school of its kind to offer women a chance to become doctors. Women flocked from all over the world for the opportunity to learn, conduct research, and teach in a hospital setting.

Then it was on to the New York Post-Graduate Medical School and Hospital for more advanced studies in a rapidly changing field. By the time she returned to Nevada, the girl who had dreamed of one day becoming a doctor had come a long way.

By 1892, Dr. Cook was trying her hand at practicing medicine in economically booming Reno. She set up an office in the two-story Golden Eagle Hotel, one of the bustling city's most popular establishments. It was a bold move made even more so after she placed an advertisement for her new practice in the *Reno Gazette-Journal*: "Dr. Eliza Cook may be consulted at her office in rooms 25 and 26 at the Golden Eagle Hotel between the hours of 9:30 to 11:30 A.M. and from 2 to 4 o'clock P.M." The newspaper advertisement itself raised eyebrows. Women physicians were rare, and one confident enough to advertise her services to some bordered on scandal.

Dr. Cook became an advocate for women in the medical profession and contributed articles to professional journals on the subject. One printed in the

October 14, 1895, edition of the *Observer* said in part:

> The college for the medical education of women founded by the Legislature of Pennsylvania was a triumphant . . . At first sight, this seemed an extraordinary proceeding and quite a startling novelty. But there remain sufficient grounds for women to pursue careers in medicine and succeed in the field. . . . Looking at the profession of female doctor, "there is nothing unreasonable in it, but the contrary, however much it may be at variance with existing usages.". . . There are now a growing number of women throughout the world in extensive practice, who have even been in difficult cases, called in by medical men themselves, in consultations. These ladies command a high degree of respect and maintain a high social status.

As the nineteenth century drew nearer to ending, women increasingly raised their collective voice as they pushed to gain the right to vote in elections, a movement known as suffrage. Although it would be many years before Nevada women secured that right, Dr. Cook was an early advocate and leader for women's suffrage.

After seeing the ravages of alcohol abuse, Dr. Cook became a vocal supporter of the temperance movement, which sought to prohibit the sale and use

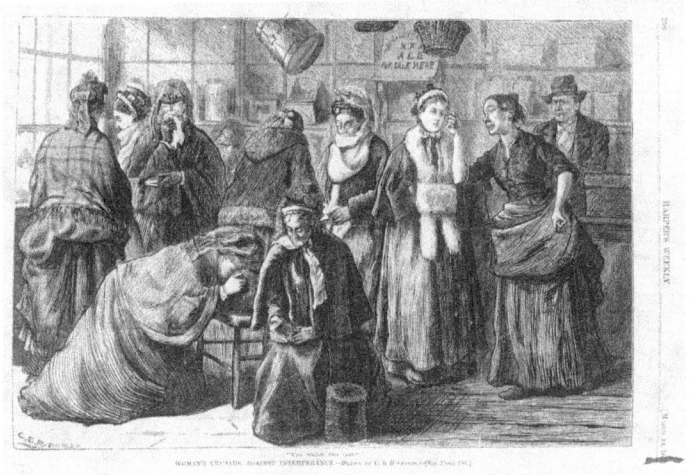

Harpers Weekly published drawings like these which depicted women in barrooms protesting the sale of alcoholic beverages. These protests influenced the temperance movement that led to Prohibition.

of liquor. She joined the local chapter of the Women's Christian Temperance Movement and for several years was its leading voice, writing about the ills wrought by alcohol in local newspapers.

The nation's temperance movement eventually prevailed in the 1919 passage of the Eighteenth Amendment to the US Constitution, which prohibited "the manufacture, sale, or transportation of intoxicating liquors." But the new law of the land proved controversial and ineffective and was repealed by ratification of the Twenty-first Amendment in 1933.

Although Reno offered the possibility of making more money, her heart had always been in the Carson

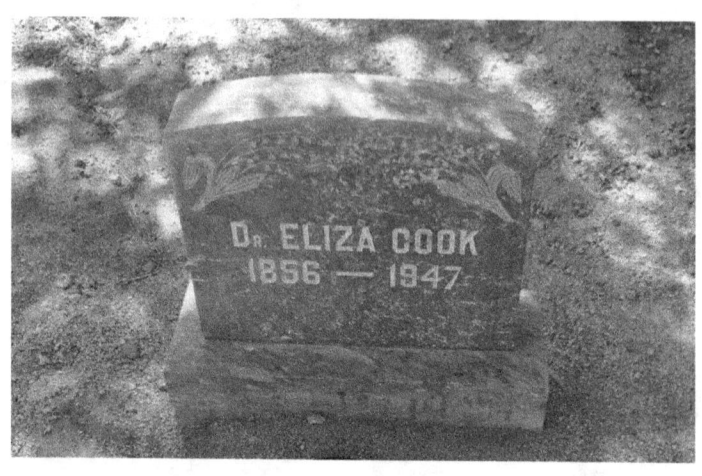

Valley. Dr. Cook returned to practice there the rest of her long career, which ended in 1922, and spent the remainder of her life in the shadow of the Sierra Nevada, tending to her patients, gardening, and reading.

When Dr. Eliza Cook died on October 2, 1947, at her Genoa home at age 91, she was a beloved figure in Northern Nevada and commonly referred to as the state's first woman physician. It had become a widely held belief, and she was proud of the unofficial title.

Although she was indeed the first female licensed in 1899 following the creation of the State Board of Medical Examiners, a more careful look at the historical record by Dr. Anton P. Sohn found at least a dozen women who practiced medicine in Nevada's boomtowns before she first started treating patients in 1884. Some of those physicians appear to have been unlicensed and may have been doctors in name only, but others touted their medical training. They specialized in treating women and children, sometimes advertised their services in the local newspapers, and were often referred to as "doctress."

In the end, it doesn't really matter whether Dr. Eliza Cook was Nevada's first female physician. Of greater importance is the lesson her life offers: by pursuing her youthful passion for medicine, she provided needed treatment to a generation of patients and saw her childhood dream come true.

6

Treating All People

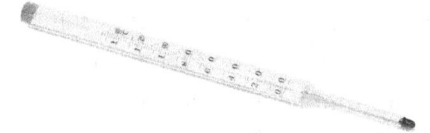

In today's world, doctors have a legal obligation to treat the patient in front of them regardless of race, gender, citizenship, or ability to pay. That wasn't always the case.

Although racial minorities struggled mightily to gain equal treatment on the frontier, W. H. C. Stephenson became known as the first Black physician in Nevada not long after the discovery of silver near Virginia City. Born in Washington, DC, in 1825, he was trained at Eclectic Institutes of Philadelphia and moved to Northern Nevada near the end of the Civil War. He treated all races and played an important role in early politics and civil rights in Nevada by encouraging Blacks to vote, a right denied until 1865 with the passage of the Fifteenth Amendment. Dr. Stephenson is believed to have died in 1899 though some sources believe he died in 1873.

Medical educations varied widely on the frontier. Born in 1844 in Illinois, Lemuel Lee served in the Union Army during the Civil War. After the war, he pursued an education at an herbal-based medical school. After graduation, he headed west to the

booming Nevada mining town of
Pioche in 1870. Although fortune
in the high-grade silver mines
proved elusive, he honed his
medical practice in Pioche before
moving to Carson City in 1879.

Lee devoted part of his
medical life to research and
recorded the vital statistics of the
community—births, deaths, ages,
and illnesses of the residents.
He was also active in party politics and performed
community services.

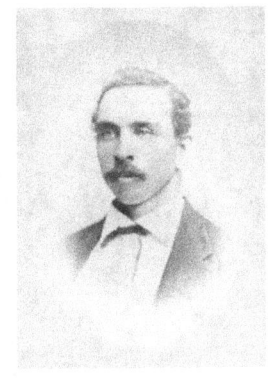

W. H. C. Stephenson

Unlike many physicians of his time, Lee treated
Native Americans. He is believed to have been the
first white doctor to deliver an Indian baby. He also
treated others afflicted with illness, and in one account
performed a needed amputation.

He was accepted by other doctors and eventually
was named president of the state Board of Health.
He was secretary of the first board of State Medical
Examiners when it was created in 1899. He died in
Carson City in 1927, and his obituary called Lee "one
of the best known physicians in Nevada."

As medicine developed and became more
specialized, doctors brought new training and skills to
Nevada. For example, Dr. Anthony Huffaker came to
Carson City after graduating from Cooper Medical
College in San Francisco and was the first licensed

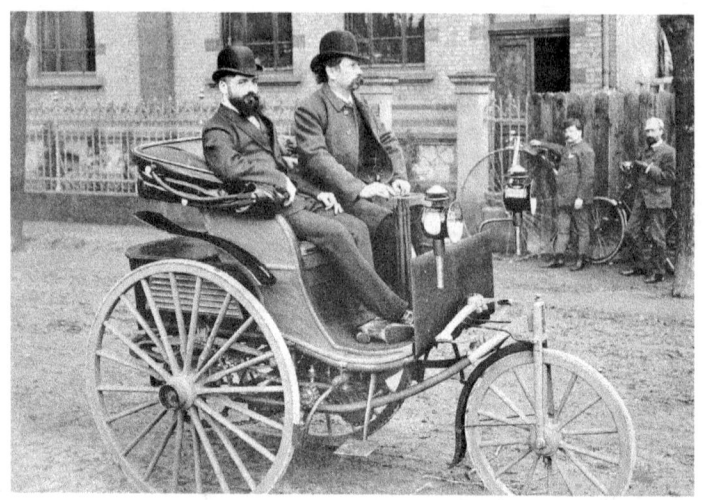

Carl Benz drives his patent motor car of 1887, an advanced version of the first motor car he invented in 1886.

pediatrician in the state. He later was named president of the Nevada State Medical Association.

While doctors in early Nevada commonly made house calls on horseback or horse-drawn carriage, the invention and mass manufacturing of the automobile sped their rounds. This led to a humorous moment for Dr. Huffaker, who had not closely studied the operator's manual for his vehicle before embarking on his patient visits, according to the Nevada Historical Society.

He returned later to his house and drove past time and again until he caught his wife's attention. The doctor shouted, "Go get the instruction booklet and throw it to me the next time around. I've forgotten how it says to stop the blamed machine!"

Around the turn of the twentieth century, Dr. Edward Shepard Grigsby brought his education from the Hahnemann Medical College in Philadelphia to Nevada after traveling as far north as Nome, Alaska. He seems to have liked living and working around mining boomtowns, for he practiced medicine in Nevada in Bullfrog, Rhyolite, and Tonopah in partnership with Dr. Patrick McDonnell.

Dr. Grigsby is remembered not for his medical expertise, but for telling friends about the time he was in Skidoo, California, outside Death Valley following a public hanging. He said he had intended to attend the event but was delayed. The townspeople obliged him by re-enacting the hanging for his benefit.

Other Nevada physicians are remembered more professionally. In the early days of Las Vegas, Dr. Halle Hewetson established a highly successful practice. That success encouraged others to study medicine and to open their own practices in Southern Nevada.

Following Hewetson's lead, Dr. Roy Martin opened a practice in the bustling railroad town as it approached the dawn of a new era of legalized gambling and a booming economy. Like Hewetson, Martin played an integral role in expanding medical services in the community. He also was an entrepreneur who speculated in the mines in the region.

7

Surviving the Great Influenza

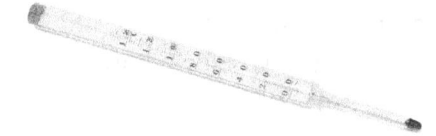

Young Edwin Cantlon would always remember the day he realized the great influenza of 1918 had finally reached Nevada. Although Edwin thought more about being a cowboy than going to school, a sudden visit to the family's Wadsworth ranch from Dr. Samuel L. Joslin grabbed the seven-year-old's full attention.

What the newspapers commonly called "the Spanish flu," out of the mistaken belief that the deadly virus had originated in that country, was a mystery even to leading medical experts as it spread rapidly across the United States and Europe. The influenza attacked the lungs and spread swiftly when an infected person coughed, sneezed, or spoke without wearing a face covering. There was no vaccine or proven treatment. By October, it had finally reached Reno and Carson City.

With about 80,000 residents, Nevada was the least densely populated state in the nation. But the flu was so contagious that it was only a matter of time before it reached even the most remote areas of the state. Nevada governor Emmet Boyle and members of the Nevada State Board of Health had surmised

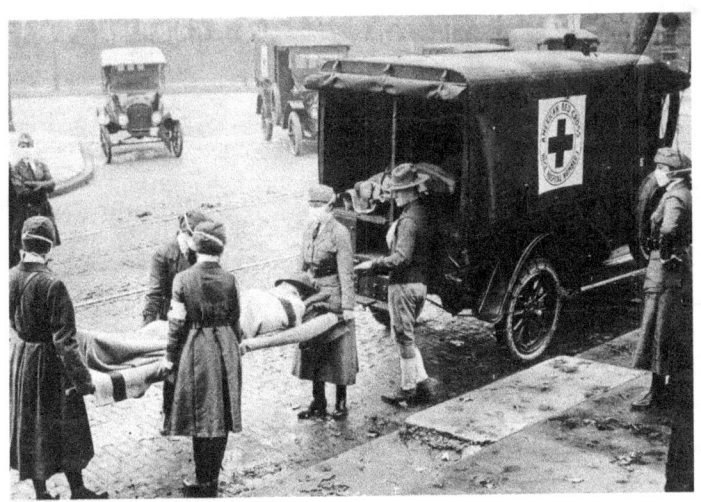

Red Cross Motor Corps during the influenza epidemic in St. Louis, Mo. in October of 1918.

that infected train passengers from San Francisco had spread it to Nevada. Although the state's first official recorded case of influenza was October 1, reporting across Nevada's vast expanse was far from accurate.

Dr. Joslin had been trained at Harvard Medical School, but nothing in his education prepared him to solve the mystery of the disease. He could only give the best medical advice available.

"Dr. Joslin passed out masks which were similar to the early-day cloth masks used in the operating room and gave the instructions to soak these masks in rubbing alcohol and then wear them over your nose and mouth," Cantlon recalled many years later. "This proved to be a chore that was beyond most people,

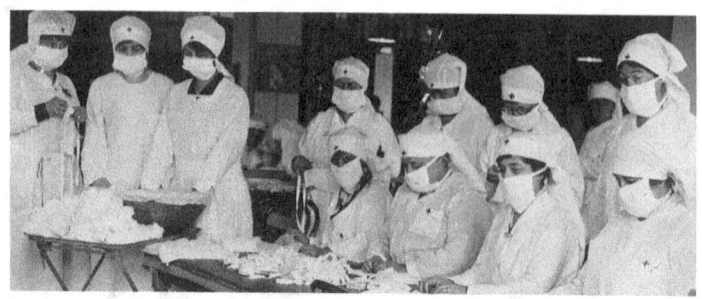

All medical personnel wore cloth masks while working with patients and medical supplies.

and the smell of the rubbing alcohol, I guess, was the deciding factor, and this was soon discarded."

After receiving instructions from the doctor, Cantlon preferred to return to playing cowboy. He'd learned to saddle a horse at age six on the family ranch, located a long and bumpy ride outside their Sparks home, and was skilled enough with a lasso to be able to help move cattle. But he soon found the spreading influenza epidemic had changed everything.

"During the epidemic, schools in Sparks were shut down for a month or so during the winter months," he recalled. "When I went back to school, two of our classmates had passed on, but my family was spared. None of our family got the flu."

Edwin Cantlon was fortunate. As the staggering loss of human life was tallied, he would one day realize just how blessed his family had been. The great influenza, which lasted through much of 1918 in the waning days of World War I and well into 1919, killed as many as seven hundred thousand Americans. It infected approximately five hundred million people worldwide—about one-third of the earth's population at the time—and led to the deaths of as many as fifty million.

Although there are distinct differences between the influenza of 1918 and the devastating coronavirus pandemic of 2020 and 2021, the similarities are instructive and the historical context can help us appreciate at least some of what Nevadans more than one hundred years ago endured. Even with a rapid response to the COVID-19 virus outbreak, and effective vaccines developed in record time, the United States still saw more than a million deaths related to the disease. Nevada paid its own terrible price with more than 10,800 as of June 2022.

Contrary to popular belief, the influenza of 1918 started not in Spain, but at a US Army camp in Funston, Kansas. A camp cook contracted the disease in March. It spread through the large temporary training base set up to prepare thousands of American troops for deployment in the battle that raged in Europe. When those troops were transported by ship to Europe to serve their country, they carried the disease with them. It swiftly spread across Europe and afflicted allies and enemies alike. No one was immune, and there was no known medical treatment or vaccine, which helps protect the body against a viral disease. (The first microscope capable of even seeing the virus wasn't developed until the early 1930s.) At the time,

DIVISION OF SANITATION
CIRCULAR NO. 1

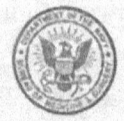

No. 130212-O

WASHINGTON, D. C., *September 20, 1918.*

INFLUENZA.

Influenza is "grippe." It is now spreading over the country in epidemic form. The last extensive epidemic occurred in 1889-90, and the disease was very prevalent for several years after.

The present epidemic disease is plain influenza. The term "Spanish influenza" has been applied because of its recent prevalence in Spain. Influenza occurs every year in the United States, but it is more contagious during an epidemic, and pneumonia is a more frequent complication.

Influenza is caused by a germ, the *influenza bacillus*, which lives but a short time outside of the body. Fresh air and sunshine kill the germ in a few minutes.

The disease is spread by the moist secretions from the noses and throats of infected persons.

Protect yourself from infection, keep well, and do not get hysterical over the epidemic.

Avoid being sprayed by the nose and throat secretions of others.

Beware of those who are coughing and sneezing.

Avoid crowded street cars—walk to the office if possible.

Keep out of crowds—avoid theaters, moving-picture shows, and other places of public assembly.

Do not travel by railroad unless absolutely necessary.

Do not drink from glasses or cups which have been used by others unless you are sure they have been thoroughly cleansed.

You can do much to lessen the danger to yourself by keeping in good physical condition.

Avoid close, stuffy, and poorly ventilated rooms—insist upon fresh air, but avoid disagreeable drafts.

Eat simple, nourishing food and drink plenty of water. Avoid constipation.

Secure at least seven hours sleep. Avoid physical fatigue.

Do not sleep or sit around in damp clothing.

Keep the feet dry.

Influenza usually has a sudden onset with chilliness, severe headache, and "aching all over." At times the disease begins with nausea, vomiting, and abdominal pain. Fever begins early. Frequently catarrhal symptoms do not appear until later. When they do they are the symptoms of a bad cold in the head with a raw throat and dry cough. Weakness and prostration out of proportion to the fever are common. Former epidemics have been characterized by marked mental depression. In the present epidemic many of the cases are having a gradual onset—more like a gradually increasing cold in the head.

Practically, the great danger from influenza is pneumonia, which tends to follow in a considerable percentage of the cases.

For the protection of others, if you are really sick stay at home and remain there until the fever is over. A day in bed at the very beginning may also save you from serious consequences later on.

If you are up and about, protect healthy persons from infection—don't spray others with the secretions from your nose and throat in coughing, sneezing, laughing, or talking. Cover the mouth with a handkerchief. Boil your handkerchiefs and other contaminated articles. Wash your hands frequently. Keep away from others as much as possible while you have a cough.

If you become ill don't try to keep on with your work. Fight the disease rationally and do not become unduly alarmed. In the average case recovery from acute symptoms follows in five or six days. To hasten recovery and lessen the danger of complications, go to bed at once and keep the body warm. There should be plenty of fresh air, but chilling is to be avoided. At the beginning of the disease a cathartic, such as 2½ or 3 grains of calomel, followed by a seidlitz powder or epsom salts, is useful. Aspirin in 5 grain doses is useful for pain, but do not take large doses of aspirin, phenacetin, or other medicines. Send for the doctor.

The Navy tried to prevent the spread of influenza by educating sailors about protecting themselves. These recommendations have not changed dramatically in one hundred years.

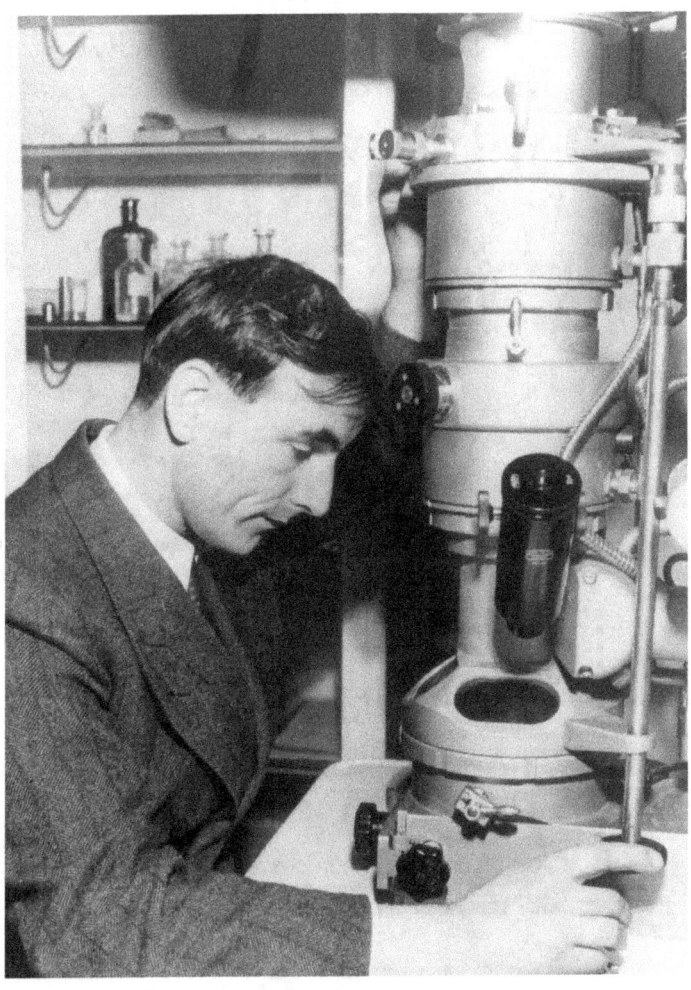

The transmission electron microscope (TEM) was invented in the early 1930s by Ernst Ruska in Germany. It dramatically improved the resolution over optical microscopes and allowed scientists to see items as small as an atom.

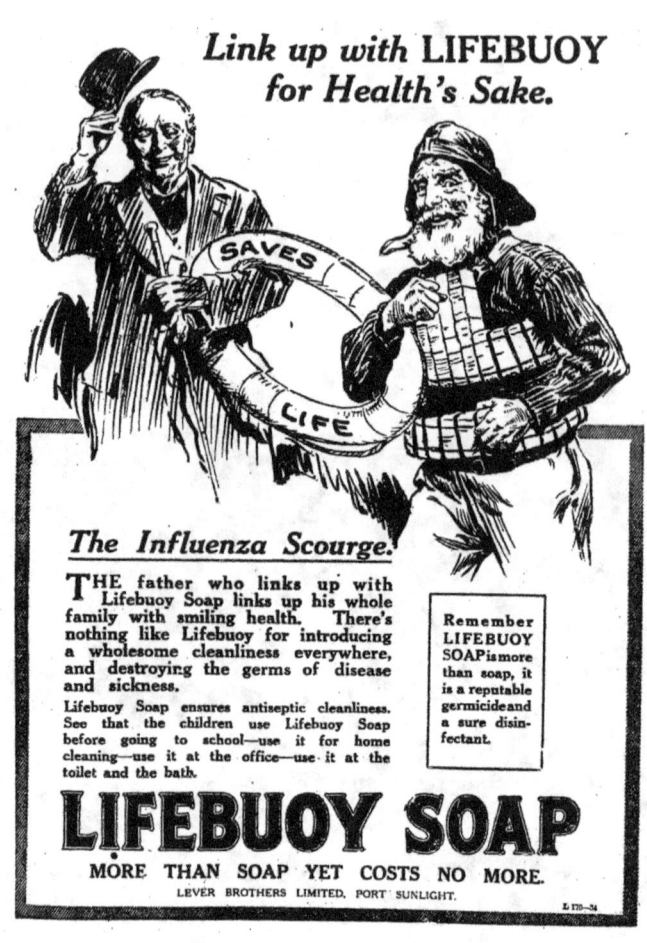

As more people died of influenza, advertising changed to remind people that even basic things like soap helped fight the spread of the disease.

the best medical experts knew little about the origin and makeup of the influenza. That is why it was so important to take the best precautions available.

The best medical practice available was wearing a face covering, practicing social spacing from one person to another, and vigorous handwashing. Those who showed signs of illness were separated from the healthy in a practice called quarantining. It wasn't a cure, but it worked to slow the spread of the disease—as long as communities were vigilant. Not all were. Confusion, disbelief, and denial were common.

Across the United States, some major cities went into lockdown. Citizens were ordered to wear masks and sometimes faced penalties if they refused. Schools and businesses were closed. Hospitals were overwhelmed. The call for volunteers and every available person with medical training went out. Tragically, the death toll increased at a blinding pace.

In Nevada, the influenza quickly spread from Reno throughout Washoe County. Officials ordered the closure of Reno High School as well as churches, theaters, and saloons. At the city's Board of Health, Dr. M. A. Robinson was adamant about the need for community compliance, telling the *Reno Evening Gazette*, "Precautions must be taken and everyone is asked to cooperate with the health authorities in keeping the disease from spreading."

Unfortunately, not everyone listened.

It wasn't long before the influenza spread from Reno to Las Vegas. As the numbers of cases climbed, Reno went into quarantine. Gardnerville and Ely followed. Other towns limited travel, banned public gatherings, and shuttered services. Children were prohibited from gathering on playgrounds. With hospital bed space extremely limited, newspapers reported that temporary hospitals were being set up in hotels, schools, and even Elks lodges.

In Southern Nevada, a headline on the front page of an early November edition of the *Las Vegas Age* reported, "Influenza Situation Becomes More Serious." Physician Roy W. Martin was the community's most respected medical professional. A chief surgeon for the Las Vegas & Tonopah Railroad, Martin founded a hospital in Las Vegas. He had experience with contagious diseases, having spent a year Monterey, California, treating patients suffering from yellow fever. After succeeding Southern Nevada's first physician, Dr. Halle Hewetson, Martin spent a four-decade career treating patients, investing in the community, and opening hospitals to meet the needs of rapidly expanding Las Vegas.

Just a year earlier, Martin had moved into the Palace Hotel on North Second Street, the first two-story building in Las Vegas, and transformed it into Las Vegas General Hospital. It would be put to good use during the influenza epidemic.

Martin had a strong message for the community published in the November 9 edition of the *Las Vegas Age*: "We are in the midst of an influenza epidemic which has been sweeping the country for several weeks. It must be controlled, or a great loss of life will result. The public must cooperate and observe the regulations of

QUARANTINE TO PREVENT SPREAD OF INFLUENZA STARTS TOMORROW

Churches and Theatres Must Close; No Public Meetings To Be Held; High School Is Closed for Week

Reno began quarantine measures to stop the flu!

the Health Department, or little will be accomplished. If you do your duty you will have but little to fear."

He followed with a list of "dos and don'ts," including wearing a face mask, increasing hygiene practices, isolating from those who show symptoms of the influenza, refraining from gathering in crowds and maintaining a social distance from others.

"The success of this campaign against influenza depends upon your co-operation," he wrote. "Intelligent people will—others must cooperate. We ask your assistance in enforcing the regulations."

There was good reason for his concern. Las Vegas, a town of about two thousand in 1918, recorded 125 influenza cases and twelve deaths related to the disease in a single week in early November. In all, at least forty deaths caused by influenza were recorded.

Nevada's small towns paid a high price, too, with deaths attributed to the flu coming in Fallon, Elko, Ely, and elsewhere. In Tonopah during the second weekend of November, nine people died from the disease.

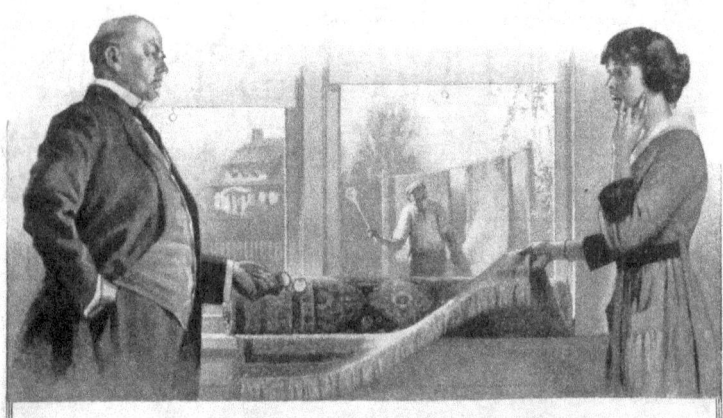

Formaldehyde is a toxic substance that causes eye, nose, and throat irritation along with headaches and rashes but people were desperate to feel safe and advertisers took advantage of that fear.

In Europe, World War I was winding down as Germany signed a formal agreement to stop fighting called an armistice treaty. Almost 117,000 American soldiers were killed in battle during the war. At home, more than 550,000 citizens lost their lives to the influenza. Nevada would record four thousand confirmed cases of influenza with the actual number likely higher.

"One can see that confusion and panic was the order of the day during the epidemic," Nevada medical historian Dr. Anton Sohn wrote in an essay on the great influenza. "The flu pandemic of 1918 is remembered in this country as much as is the horror of World War I. We can readily understand the concern of Nevadans in 1918, if we consider that deaths due to influenza where the cause of the disease was unknown, and it outnumbered our combat fatalities."

Although newspapers commonly called for the public to remain calm, there appeared no end in sight. Tales of devastated neighborhoods and whole families falling to the disease only increased anxiety. More damaging were calls from some public officials to take precautions but practice "business as usual." Nevada's Board of Health, which was having difficulty keeping up with an accurate count of the sick and deceased, wrote that "no matter what the cause of the disease or the course of treatment pursued, there can be no question or doubt but that 'fear' should have been entered in the death certificate as the remote cause of death."

With no known cure, and fear rising, some people chose to rely on folk remedies to protect them from the flu. As Nevada historian Phillip I. Earl discovered, some well-meaning people believed carrying a potato in each pocket would ward off the mysterious killer. Others relied on eating "red pepper sandwiches." Still others thought sprinkling sulfur in their shoes would do the trick. Sulfur, a stinky chemical, was used as a disinfectant.

Fear took its toll, and experiences not rooted in fact enflamed people's anxieties. As John M. Barry wrote in his book *The Great Influenza*, "The strongest weapon against pandemic is the truth." Following the facts, as best they are known, is the only way to overcome the fear associated with diseases that appear so mysterious and even supernatural.

Amid the pandemic, Carson City physician Ernst Krebs noticed that for some reason members of the region's Washoe tribe weren't hit as hard by the virus that was sweeping through the land and killing thousands from big cities and isolated small towns. They weren't immune to the disease, exactly, but those who were afflicted appeared to recover more quickly. And, he observed, none died from the virus.

At the Western Shoshone Agency, official headquarters of the tribe in the state, members were ordered to only go to the store when necessary. As a precaution, transactions took place on the porch outside the store.

"Owing to cases of Spanish Influenza on the reservation," Superintendent H. D. Lawshe wrote, "everyone is cautioned to take every care that they do not expose themselves or their neighbors."

Other Native Americans weren't as fortunate. Their misery was well documented because the federal government supervised Indian reservations through the Bureau of Indian Affairs. At the Reno Indian Agency, a photographer captured the conditions the Paiute faced as the influenza spread through Virginia City. "In this shack," an agent wrote in a note accompanying the photograph, "I found four people laying on the dirt floor in rags apparently all suffering from influenza. I was told that they had refused medicine from the white doctor and Dick Mauwee, a Paiute enrolled at Pyramid Lake reservation, was the doctor."

For all the pain, suffering, and death caused by the great influenza of 1918, its challenges also served to inspire a new generation of medical professionals who experienced firsthand the need for improving health services to their fellow citizens. Young Edwin Cantlon was part of that generation. Although he embraced the cowboy way of life once common in western Nevada, he followed his brother Vernon's lead and pursued a career in medicine. With his public-school education and degree from the University of Nevada, he was accepted into and excelled at Harvard University's medical and surgical

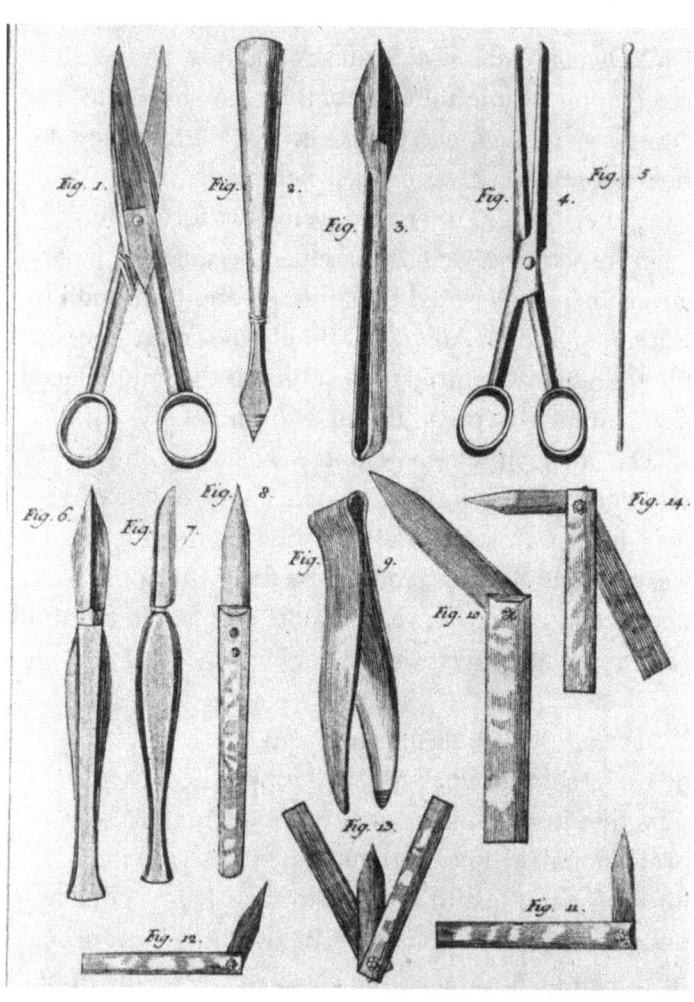

Some tools such as these knives that doctors used in the 1800s for bloodletting haven't changed dramatically in hundreds of years, but even minor changes have improved every aspect of medical care.

programs. He also served four years as a military surgeon during World War II.

When he returned from the war, the boy who had experienced the pandemic opened a private surgical practice and, along with brother Vernon, helped raise the professional standards of physicians in Northern Nevada by establishing the Reno Surgical Society. A cowboy at heart, he continued to ride horses. He died in 2004 after a long life spent contributing to the health and care of his fellow Nevadans.

8

In Pursuit of a Medical Education

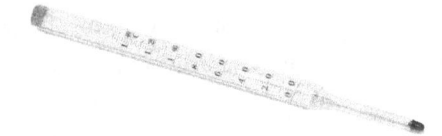

In a way, the story of medicine in Nevada ends as it began: in pursuit of the best medical treatment available. In its wild days as a territory and young state, Nevada attracted several doctors—many of whom lacked a medical education. That gradually changed as the state matured and medicine advanced from the application of home remedies to a more science-based understanding.

If Nevada's doctors and nurses were educated, they received their training from outside the state. Shortages of physicians, nurses, and other health professionals increased the need for professional training. Nursing classes such as the one started by the Catholic Sisters of St. Mary's in Virginia City eventually led to full-fledged university programs.

It took longer for Nevada to develop its own medical school. Beginning with a 1969 law that created a two-year medical training program at the University of Nevada, Reno, the state finally began to produce a new generation of doctors. By 1977, the study of medicine was expanded to a four-year program. By 1980, almost 130 years after Dr. Daggett set foot in the

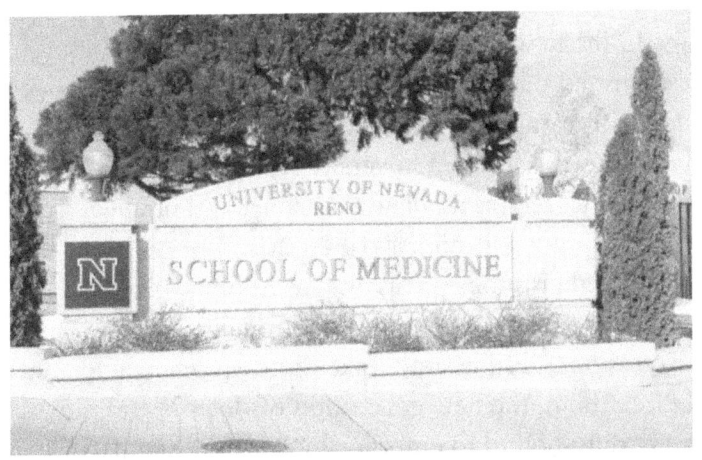

Established in 1969, UNR School of Medicine has graduated more than eighteen hundred doctors.

territory, Nevadans saw the graduation of the state's first class of physicians trained within its borders. Since then, more than eighteen hundred graduates of the program have pursued careers in family practice, internal medicine, psychiatry, and other specialties. They have participated in residencies in association with hospitals throughout Northern Nevada, many of which operate in underserved areas.

In 2014, the state received more promising news with the opening of the UNLV School of Medicine. Later named for legendary casino developer Kirk Kerkorian, the Southern Nevada medical school celebrated its first graduating class in 2021. The students received free tuition thanks to generous donations led by the Engelstad Foundation.

In the new century, private medical universities also established themselves in Nevada to meet a growing need for trained physicians and nurses. Perhaps the best known is Touro University Nevada, which in 2021 offered degrees in medicine, nursing, and physical therapy among its courses of study.

Whether public or private institutions, they all served a rapidly growing need for qualified health professionals in the state. Like those healers who came before them, the new generation of doctors and nurses were duty-bound to embrace high ethical standards and carry out the best medical practices.

Glossary

Acupuncture: Ancient Chinese medical practice that uses needles to help relieve pain and cure illness.

Herbal medicine: A practice of medicine that uses roots, stems, flowers, and the seeds of plants to treat and prevent illness.

Medicine Wheel: In Native American culture, it is used to refer to a holistic view of the physical and spiritual world around us, including references to the four directions (north, south, east, and west), the sky above, ground below, and the inner center.

Midwife: Traditionally, a woman who helps pregnant women in the months leading up to and including childbirth.

Nurse: A trained person who works with physicians and assists with patient care.

Respiratory: Referring to the breathing and the use of the lungs.

Poultice: Traditionally, a wound covering meant to protect and aid in healing.

Shaman: A spiritual leader who often also treats patients.

Traditional Chinese Medicine (TCM): A practice of medicine that uses herbal products, acupuncture, and an ancient philosophy of healing to treat illness.

Key Characters

Dr. Eliza Cook: Born in 1856 in Salt Lake City, Cook moved to Carson Valley as a young girl and assisted a local physician when she was a teenager. She later graduated from Cooper Medical College and returned to Carson Valley to begin a long career as one of the state's first female physicians. She was also active in the women's suffrage movement, which helped women win the right to vote.

Dr. Charles Daggett: Born in Vermont in 1806, Daggett graduated from Berkshire Medical College outside Boston and moved to Carson Valley in 1851. In addition to a long career in the practice of medicine, Daggett also served as the area's prosecuting attorney and tax collector and assessor.

Dr. Halle Hewetson: Born in Clairsville, Ohio, in 1864, Hewetson graduated from the University of Pennsylvania Department of Medicine in 1886. Serving as a physician for the railroad, he came to the Las Vegas townsite in 1905. He was Southern Nevada's first practicing physician and started the town's first hospital.

Dr. Anthony Huffaker: Born in 1863, Huffaker graduated from Cooper Medical College (later known as Stanford Medical School) and opened a practice in 1896 in Carson City. He was an early president of the Nevada State Medical Association.

Judge Orson Hyde: An original apostle of the Church of Jesus Christ of Latter-day Saints, Hyde was sent to the Carson Valley in 1855 to help settle the area. He was the first judge in the Utah Territory, part of which later became the state of Nevada. He later returned to Utah.

Dr. Simeon Lemuel Lee: Born in 1844, Dr. Lee graduated from an herbal medicine school in 1870 and moved to the

Nevada mining town of Pioche in 1872 before moving his practice to Carson City in 1879. He was a president of the state Board of Health and a member of the first board of State Medical Examiners when it was formed in 1899.

Dr. Royce "Roy" Wood Martin: Born in 1874 in Table Rock, Nebraska, Martin was believed to be the second practicing physician in Southern Nevada. He also dabbled in mining investments and later served as the chief surgeon for the Las Vegas & Tonopah Railroad. He was active in politics, opened a hospital, and later partnered with W. E. Ferron to open the White Cross Drug Store in downtown Las Vegas.

Florentina "Nellie" Nostrossa: Born in 1835 in Peru, she was a beloved and influential midwife and nurse in Eureka. She died in 1922.

Selected Bibliography and Further Reading

Elliott, Russell R., and William D. Rowley. *History of Nevada*, Second Edition, Revised. Lincoln: University of Nebraska Press, 1987.

Dangberg, Grace, ed. *Carson Valley: Historical Sketches of Nevada's First Settlement.* Carson City: Carson Valley Historical Society, 1972.

Geuder, Patricia A., Editor. *Pioneer Women of Nevada.* Carson City/Reno: Nevada Division of the American Association of University Women, 1976.

Green, Michael S. *Nevada: A History of the Silver State.* Reno: University of Nevada Press, 2015.

Hulse, James W. *The Silver State: Nevada's Heritage Reinterpreted.* Reno: University of Nevada Press, 1991.

Paher, Stanley W., ed., *Nevada Towns and Tales*. Las Vegas: Nevada Publishing. 1981.

Rusco, Elmer. *Good Time Coming? Black Nevadans in the Nineteenth Century.* Westport, CT: Greenwood Press, 1975.

Sohn, Anton P. *The Healers of 19th-Century Nevada.* Reno: University of Nevada, Greasewood Press, 1997

Sohn, Anton P., and Robert Daugherty. *150 Years of Nevada Medicine (And More): Nevada's Men & Women Healers.* Reno: Greasewood Press, 2014.

Train, Percy. *Medicinal Uses of Plants by Indian Tribes of Nevada.* London: Forgottenbooks.com, 2018.

Questions for Discussion

1. What made Native American medical practitioners different from some other doctors? How were they similar?

2. How were the Chinese treated in frontier Nevada?

3. Why were midwives so important on the frontier?

4. Why was the creation of medical and nursing schools important in Nevada?

5. In frontier Nevada, doctors often played more than one role. Can you name some of the other business and professional activities they participated in?

6. The great influenza of 1918 killed many people. Why was it so deadly?

7. Eliza Cook is sometimes known as Nevada's first female physician. What made her important to the development of medicine in the state?

8. Doctors Halle Hewetson and Roy Martin played important roles in the development of medicine in Southern Nevada. What did they accomplish?

9. In Nevada, UNLV and UNR each offer medical degrees. Why do you think it's important to have medical training programs in the state?

10. Do you think medical professionals should have an obligation to treat all people?

Index

A
Achilles 14, 15
acupuncture viii, 24, 61
advertisement 32, 33, 48
Atkinson, Barbara viii
Aurora vii, 20, 21
avalanche 19

B
barbers 8
Berkshire Medical College 5, 62

C
Cantlon, Dr. Edwin 42, 43, 44, 55
Central Pacific Railroad 19
Chew Kee Store 22, 23
childbirth 7, 25, 61
Chinese Exclusion Act of 1882 23
Chinese Gardens 20
Cheung, Dr. Yee Fung 22, 23
civil rights 18, 38
Civil War vii, 7, 8, 38
contagious diseases 50
Cook, Dr. Eliza v, 30, 31, 32, 33, 34, 36, 37, 62, 65
Cooper Medical College in San Francisco 39
COVID-19 45
Cowboy Bandages 16

D
Daggett, Charles vii, 2, 3, 5, 6, 8, 9, 58, 62
Daggett Pass 6
dances 11
denial 49, 51, 53
Donner Party 1

E
Eclectic Institutes of Philadelphia 38
Engelstad Foundation 59
ether 8

F
Fifteenth Amendment 38
formaldehyde 52
frostbite 1–3

G
Georgetown Trail 5
gold fields 1
Grigsby, Dr. Edward Shepard 41

H
herbs 3, 9, 10, 16, 17, 21, 61
Hewetson, Dr. Halle 41, 50, 62, 65
hot springs 10, 12
Huffaker, Dr. Anthony 39, 40, 62
Hyde, Judge Orson 1, 3, 62

I
indigenous tribes 9
indigestion 13, 15
influenza v, vii, 7, 42, 43, 44, 45, 46, 48, 49, 50, 51, 53, 54, 55, 65

J
Joslin, Dr. Samuel L. 42, 43

K
Kerkorian, Kirk viii, 59
Kingsbury Grade 6

L
Lee, Dr. Lemuel vii, 38, 62

M
John Mackay 26
Magnuson Act 23
Martin, Royce "Roy" W. 41, 65
Mauwee, Dick 55
medical masks 43, 44, 49, 51
medicine hoop 9
medicine wheel 9, 10
mesquite 12
midwives vii, 25, 28, 61, 63, 65
mint 15
mullein 16
myths 53, 54

N
Native Americans 9–16, 39, 54, 55
Nevada Board of Health 39, 53, 63
Nevada State College 29
Nevada statehood 5, 19, 26
Nevada State Medical Association 40, 62
Nellie Nostrossa vii, 25
nursing school 27, 28
nursing shortage 28, 29

O
opium 8, 23
Oxborrow, Mary vii, 25

P
Pacific Railway Acts 18
Paiute 9, 55
Pony Express ii, vii
poultice 10, 13
prayers 11

Q
quarantine 49, 51

R
Red Cross Society of Nevada 27, 43
Reno Surgical Society 57
Ruska, Ernst 47

S
San Francisco 17, 18, 31, 39, 43
shaman 11, 12, 61
Shoshone 9, 54

slaves 5
Smith, Dr. H. W. 31
Sohn, Dr. Anton P. iv, 36
Stanford University School of
    Medicine 31
State Board of Nurse
    Examiners 29
State Medical Examiners 39, 63
Stephenson, Dr. H. C. 38, 39
Stereoscopic photos 7
St. Mary's Hospital vii, 26,
    27, 28
suffrage 34, 35, 62
surgery 26, 56, 57
sweat lodge 11

T

tea 10, 12, 15, 16, 18
Tonopah 41, 50, 51, 63
Touro University Nevada 29, 60
Traditional Chinese Medicine
    17, 21, 24, 61
transmission electron
    microscope (TEM) 47
turpentine 3, 4

Twenty-first Amendment 35

U

University of Nevada School
    of Medicine vii
UNLV viii, 29, 59, 65
UNR 29, 55, 58, 59, 65
Utah Territory 1, 62

V

vaccine 42, 45

W

Washoe 9, 15, 49, 54
willow 13, 15
Women's Christian
    Temperance Movement
    35
Wongu University of Oriental
    Medicine 24
World War I 44, 53

Y

yarrow 15, 16
yucca 13

About the Author

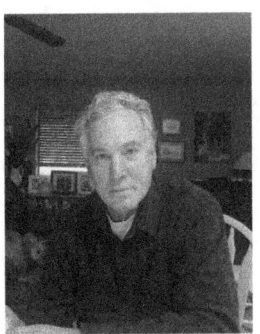

Native Nevadan John L. Smith is a longtime journalist and the author of more than a dozen books including *Saints, Sinners, and Sovereign Citizens: The Endless War Over the West's Public Lands*. He has won many state, regional, and national awards for his writing and was inducted into the Nevada Press Association Newspaper Hall of Fame in 2016, the same year that saw him honored with the James Foley/Medill Medal for Courage in Journalism, the Society of Professional Journalists Ethics Award, and the Ancil Payne Award for Ethics in Journalism from the University of Oregon. He freelances for a variety of publications, including *The Nevada Independent*. The father of a grown daughter, Amelia, he is married to the writer Sally Denton and makes his home in Boulder City, Nevada.

www.ingramcontent.com/pod-product-compliance
Lightning Source LLC
Chambersburg PA
CBHW062040120526
44592CB00035B/1696